AF365511

Going to the dentist is fun

D.D.S.M.S. Cecilia López Demerutis

Going to the dentist is fun

Second Edition
Saltillo, Coahuila 2021
D.R. Quintanilla Ediciones
Printed in Mexico
© D.D.S.M.S. Cecilia López Demerutis

quintanilla ediciones

ISBN: 978-607-9417-98-7
www.quintanillaediciones.com

Printing was completed at Quintanilla Ediciones,
with a total of 100 copies.

With love
to Liky, Ely,
and Eliseo.

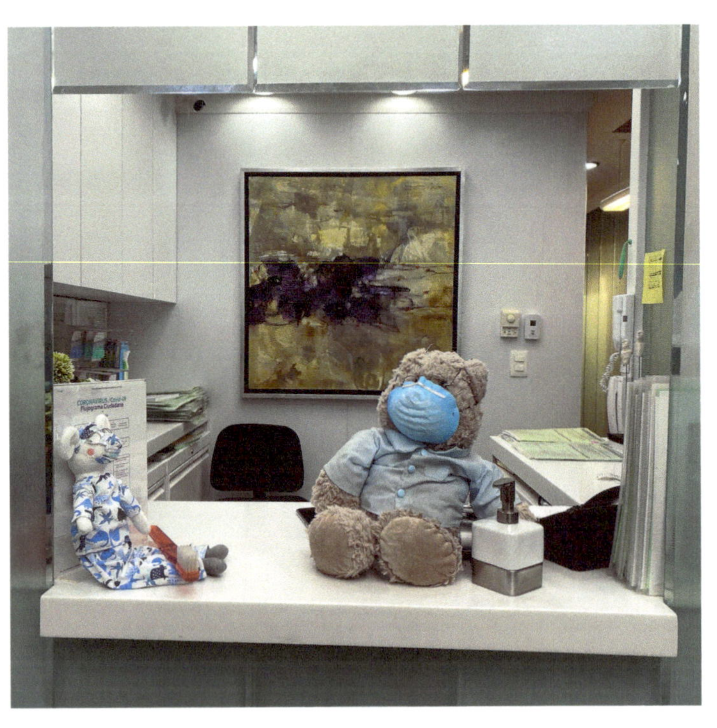

4

antiago Mouse and
Genaro Bear had their
first visit to the dentist.
At first, they were very
nervous, because they did not
know what was going to
happen, but they soon
realized that it can be an
enjoyable and healthy
experience.
C'mon! Let's join them for
their dentist's appointment.
Remember that you can
always come accompanied by
your parents or guardians.

Let's get started!!

Which flavor
do you prefer?

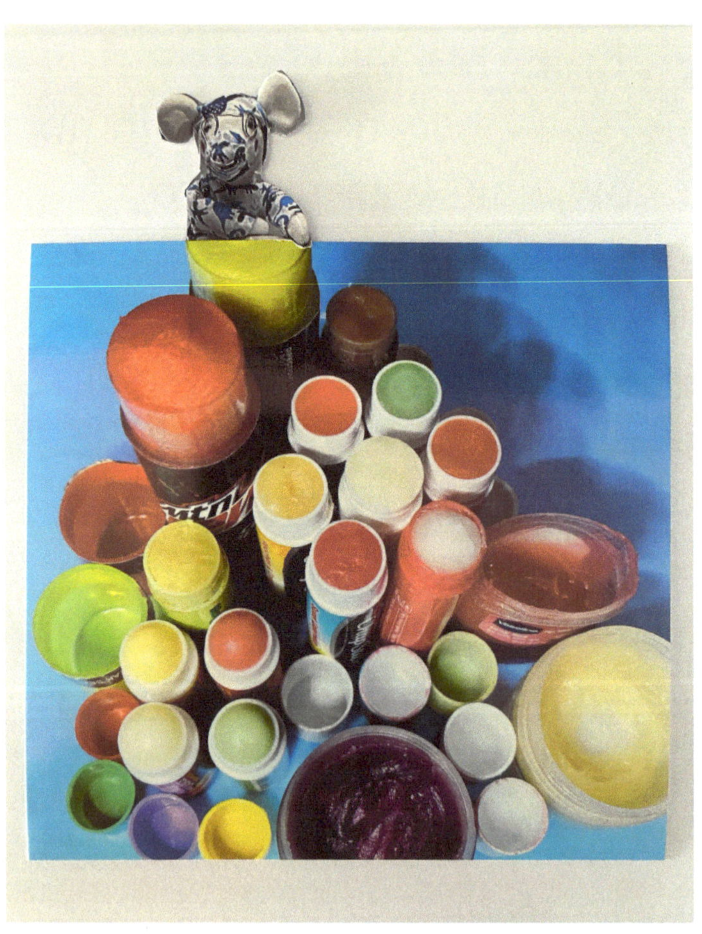

First, the dentist will explain how they will work in your mouth. It's normal that due to changes in the weather your lips could dry out or split a little. So first, the dentist will moisturize them with vaseline lip balm. You can choose from several flavors: cherry, pineapple, strawberry, mint, and many more!

Genaro Bear learned during his visit that he must brush his teeth very well every day to keep them healthy.
It is very important to always brush your teeth three times a day, after every meal.

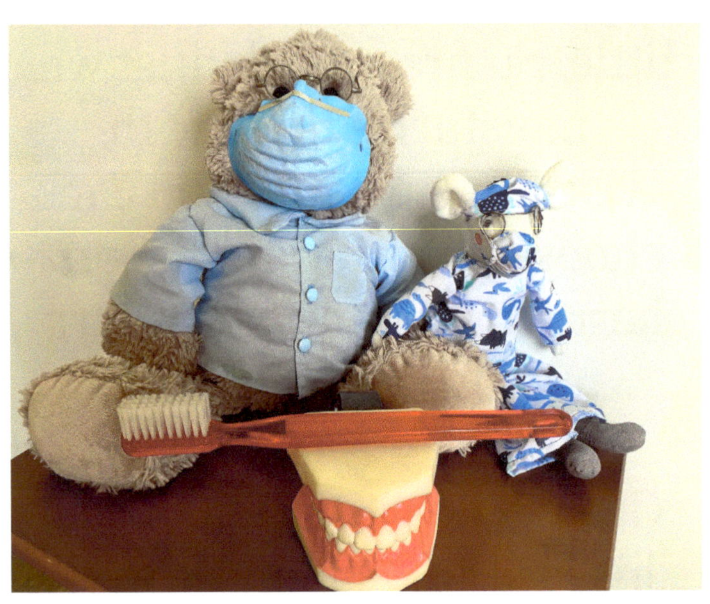

8

Here's how:

Choosing the right toothbrush
for your teeth is very
important, if you have
small teeth use a small brush.

If your teeth are a little
bigger use a medium brush. If
you are under 12 years old you
should not use electric
toothbrushes. If you are
older you can use them as
long as you are always in front
of a mirror and make sure
that you are not touching your
gums since you can hurt them.

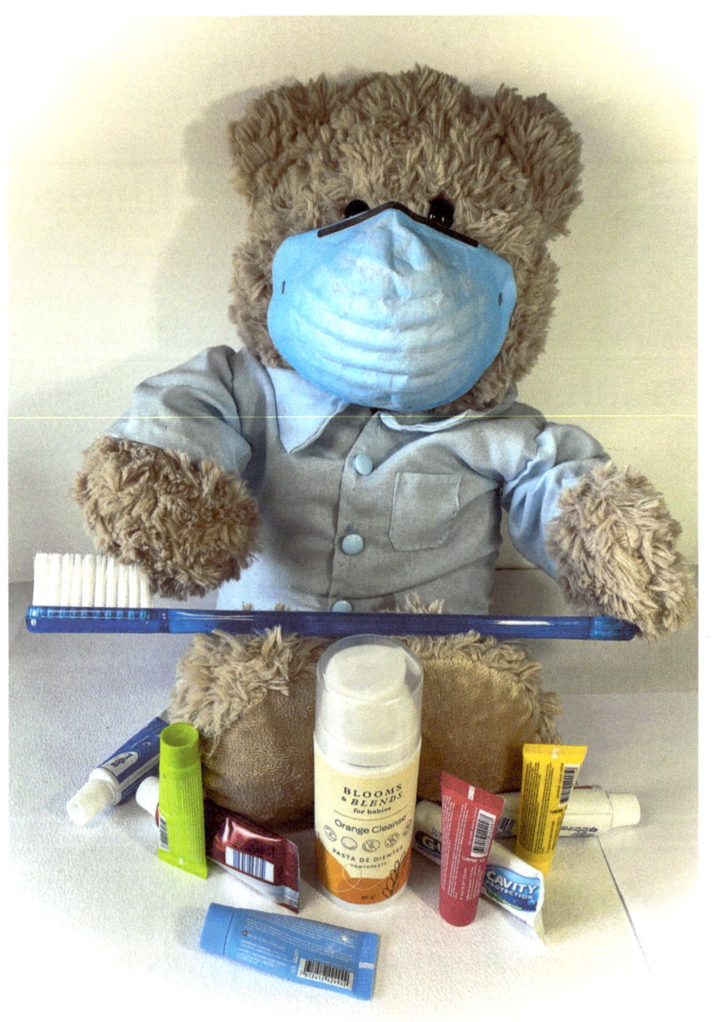

BLOOMS
& BLENDS
for babies
Orange Cleanser
PASTA DE DIENTES
TOOTHPASTE
CAVITY
PROTECTION

Toothpaste is made of soap,
adhesive, and vitamins
(fluoride). To properly brush
your teeth, the first thing you
have to do is dampen the
toothbrush with water,
then apply a little paste to the
bristles, and then start brushing
from the molars. Be mindful
that if you put the toothpaste
on the brush first and then add
water to it, the fluoride can wash
down the drain instead of
protecting your teeth.
There are many flavors and
brands of toothpastes. Choose
the one you like the most
and remember to only use
a small amount, about
the size of a pea.

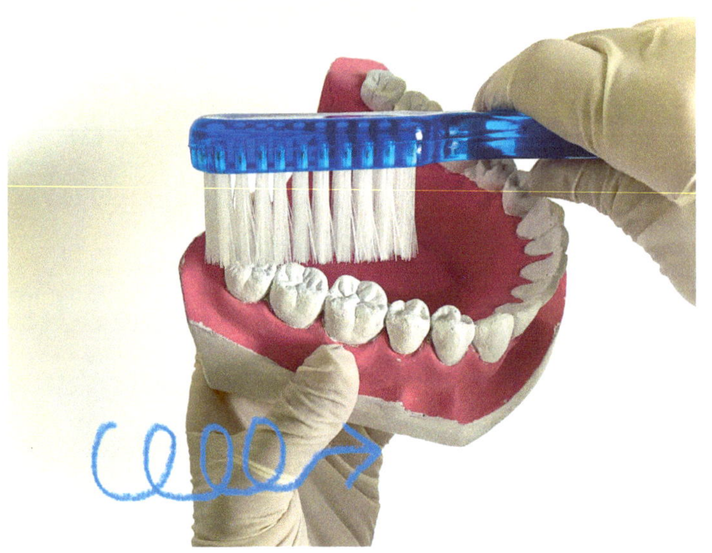

It's easy and fun
to brush your teeth!

Genaro Bear learned that we
should start brushing from
the molars, using a circular
motion to clean the part
of the teeth that we use
to chew our food.

Remember to count to '10'
when brushing each
and every area of your
mouth to ensure you
are doing an excellent job.

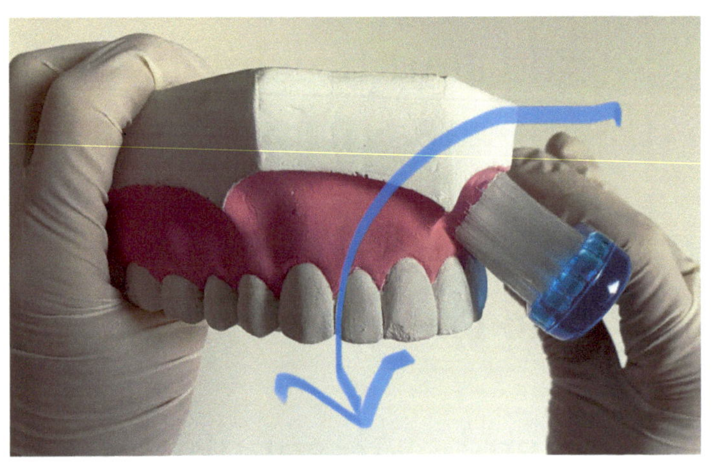

Then, very carefully,
you have to brush your front
upper teeth.

It is important to brush
these teeth from top to
bottom, front and back,
always starting from
the gums.

**You have
to repeat this process
on all your teeth.**

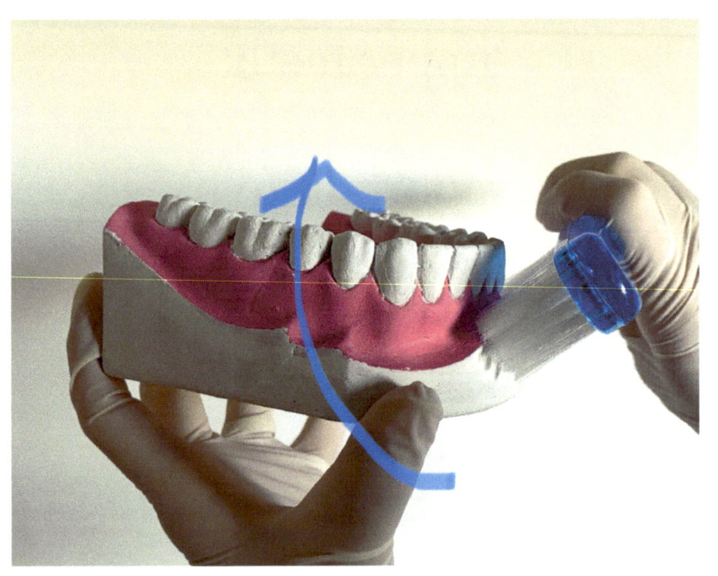

16

Your bottom teeth
should be brushed from
the bottom up, front
and back.

Repeat this 10 times
every 2 to 3 teeth.

If you notice that your gums
are red, you can get them
to change to a pinkier color
by following this technique.

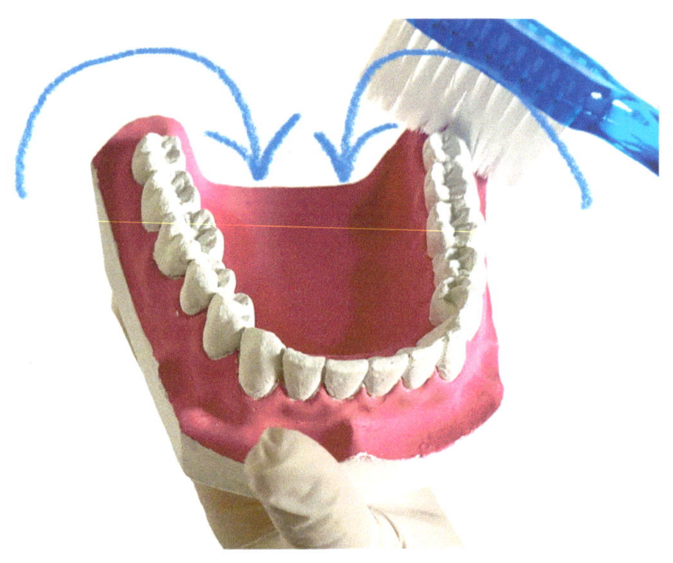

18

The back of your molars
should also be brushed.

In this area, you should
rotate the brush at least
3 times from the front
to the back of your teeth.

It is vital
to keep this area very clean
because as you grow older,
new molars will appear.

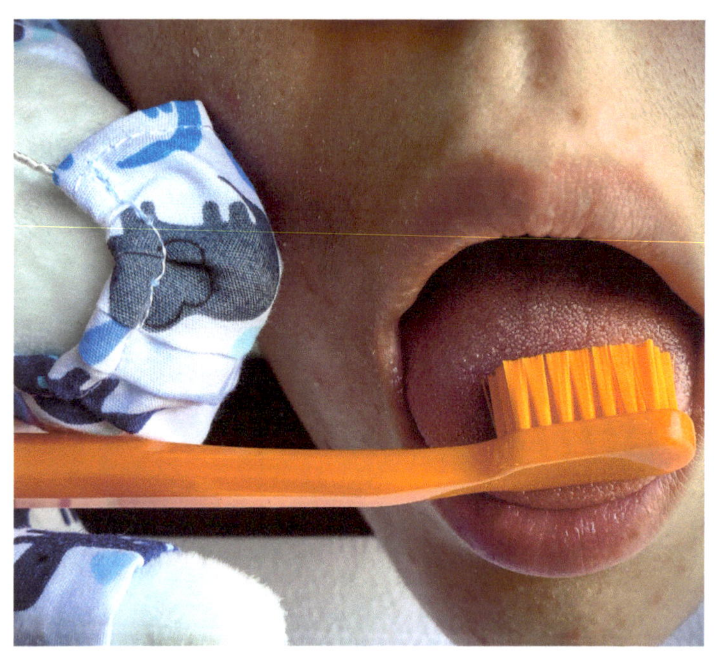

After you finish
brushing your teeth,
**you should not forget
to clean your tongue!**

You should brush it
outwardly three times.

Do it carefully and with
tenderness so it will be very
clean. If you notice your
tongue is white, you need
to drink more water.

Drink a glass of water
and you will feel better.

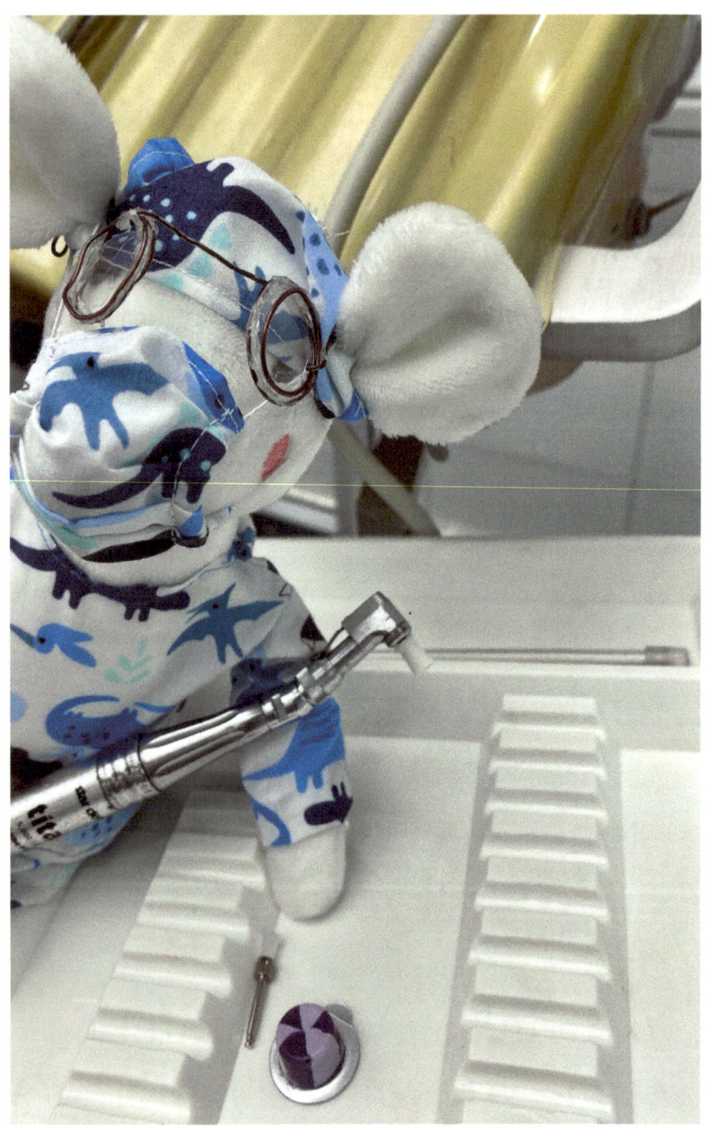

Ideally, to avoid tooth decay, your dentist will do a deep cleaning at least once or twice a year. This cleaning consists of removing the bacterial plaque (made up of food remains with tiny little bugs), tartar (build up) using a rubber cone, and a tiny rotating brush.

Then the dentist will use a cleaning paste which has different flavors such as cherry, grape, mint or vanilla ice cream. You will rinse and spit it out and then they will put a vitamin concentrate on your teeth (fluoride) so that they will be very strong.

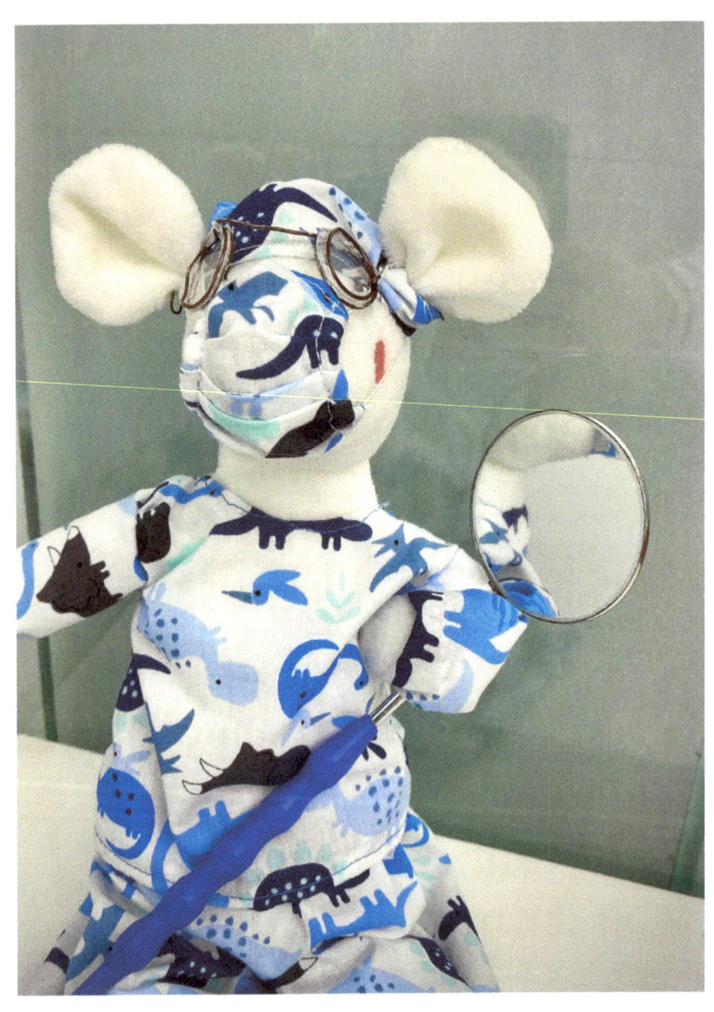

Santiago Mouse reminds
you that your dentist has
the best technology to protect
your oral health.

He and Genaro Bear feel
safer knowing what
procedures will occur and
how the dentist will carry
them out. So if you have the
curiosity of an investigator,
you can ask for a little mirror
or even bring your own
to see the work your dentist
does inside your mouth.

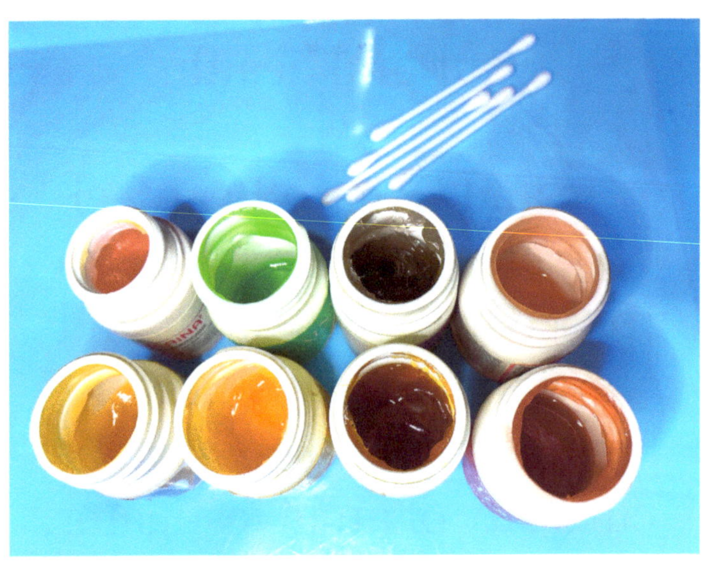

26

If the work your dentist is
doing on your tooth is not
very deep, they will put
a numbing cream on your
gums and tooth to treat you.

The cream is called
"topical anesthesia".

You can also choose from
different flavors such as
strawberry, cherry, pineapple
with coconut, mango, grape,
or banana and you might even
feel a slight tingle
on your teeth.

No harm in smiling.

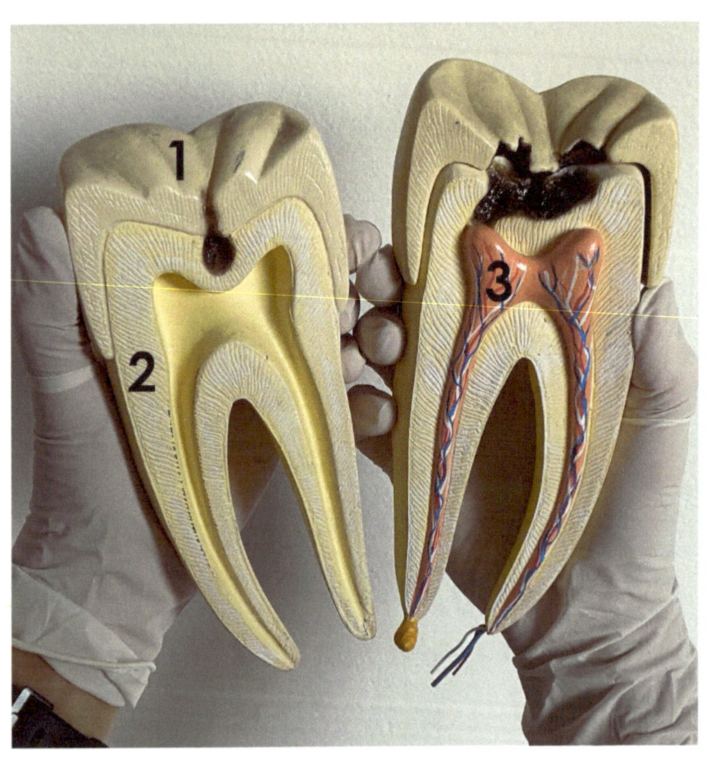

1
2
3

Teeth are very strong and are
made of three different layers:

1. Enamel:
This is the first layer.
It is white and visible in
your mouth.
2. Dentin:
The second layer is in the
middle and protects the
nerve of the tooth.
3. Pulp:
The third layer is at the
center of the tooth, within
it is the nerve, vein and
artery which like hoses
transport nutrients
to the tooth.

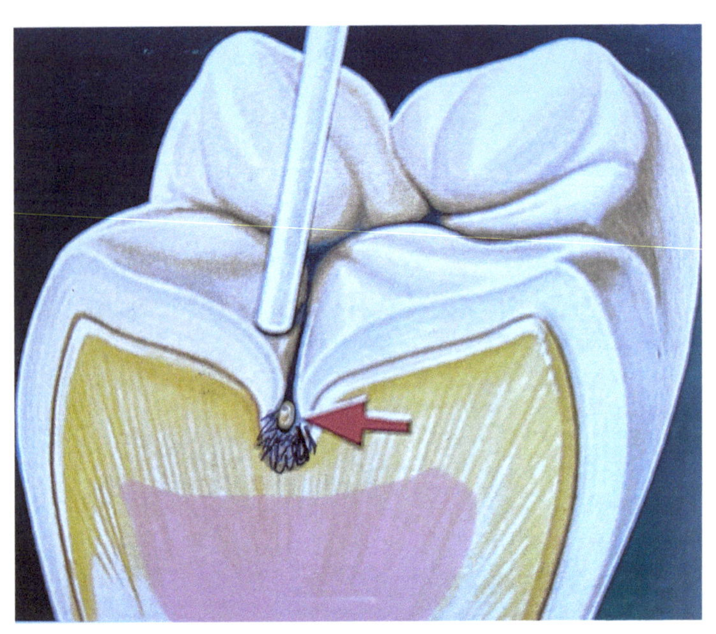

Genaro Bear also learned
about tooth decay during
his visit. The dentist told
him that cavities are
a disease that destroy teeth.

Cavities appear when you DO
NOT brush your teeth
thoroughly or when food
remains are left on your teeth
that then spoil; becoming
acidic, which leads to the
weakening of the enamel
of the tooth.

This allows the bugs to pass
through the hardest part
of the tooth, reaching the
dentin and the pulp, which
can cause pain.

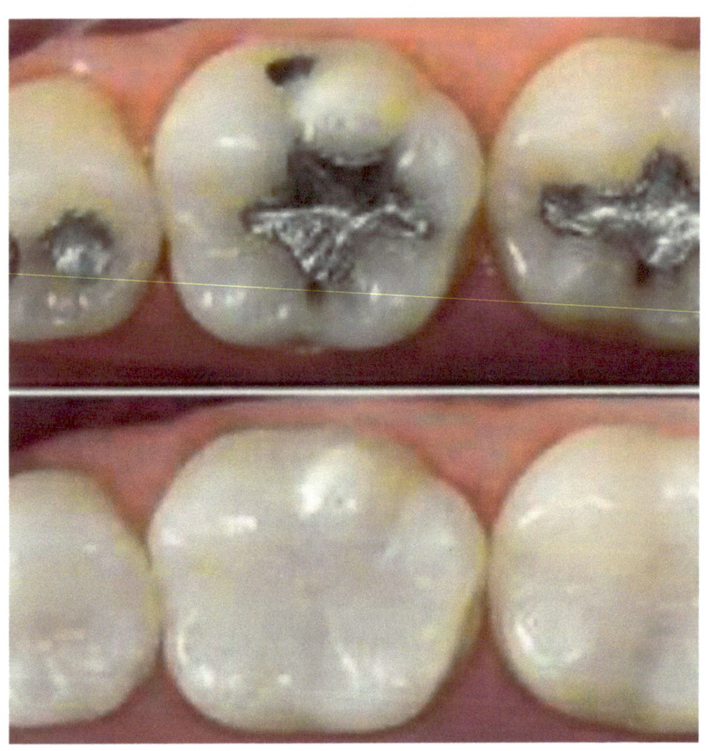

A few years ago, if a dentist had found cavities in your teeth, they would have removed and covered them with a silver material called "amalgam".

Nowadays, there are composites and sealants that when placed on the teeth help make them look healthy, white and shiny.

"And you can keep a beautiful smile".

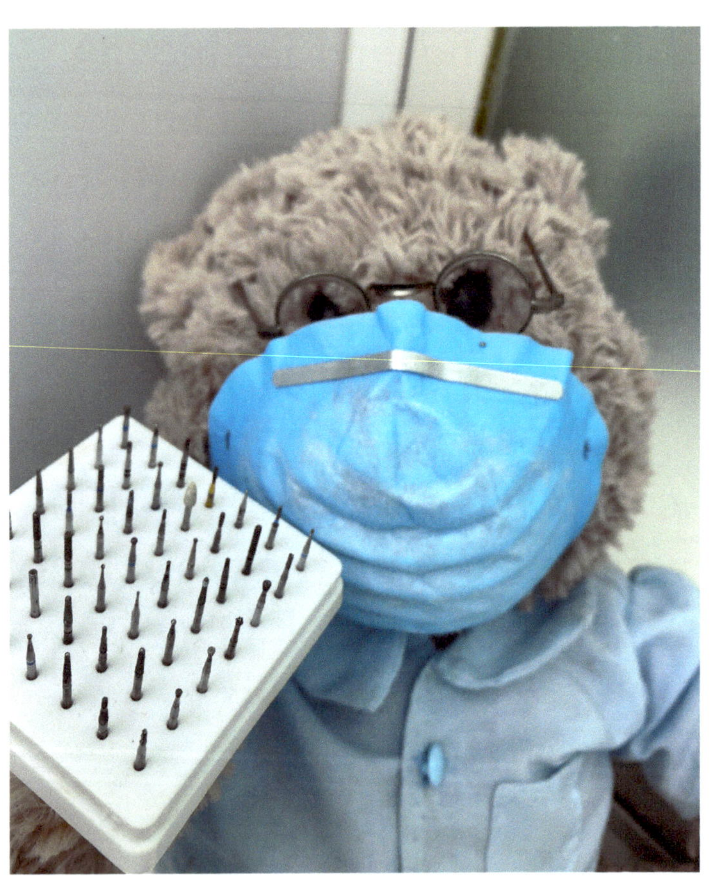

34

Today, cavities are removed
with a handpiece;
a machine that buzzes like
a bee, squirts water, and has
a circled tip called "bur"
(but it's not cold even if it
sounds like it is). "Burs"
can be made of carbon steel
or diamond, so bad bugs
can be removed with its help.

Genaro Bear shows them to
you so you can see them and
know that they don't hurt.

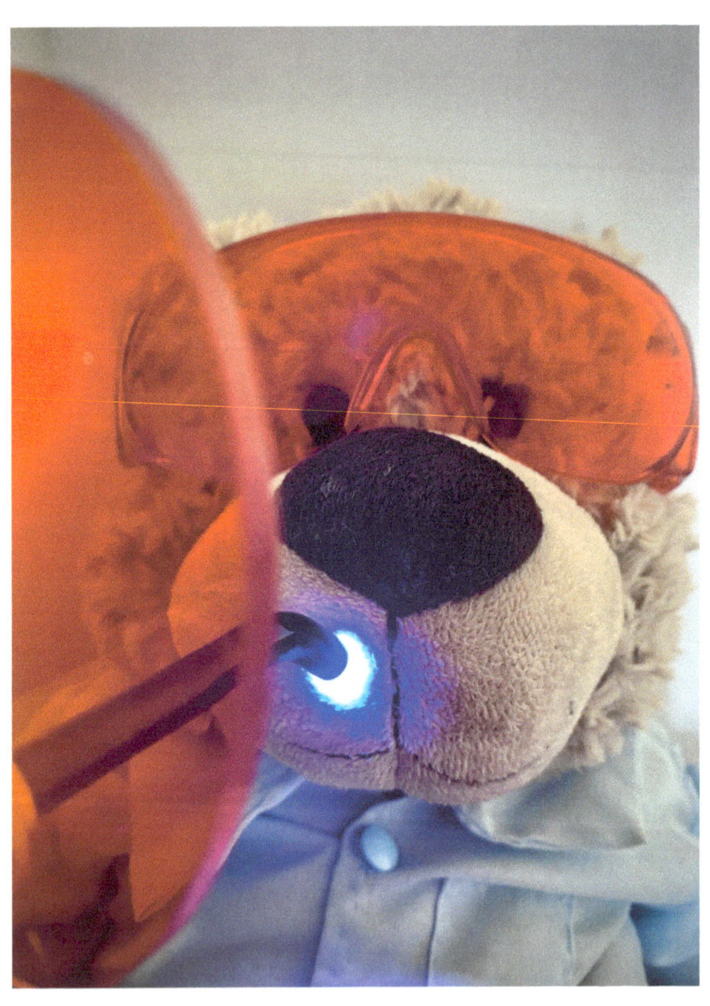

Once all the cavities
have been removed from
the tooth, the dentist will
place a material that is the
same color as your teeth
where the cavities used to be.
This material hardens with
a special light, so you'll get
to wear orange lenses
to protect your eyes.

You can tell your friends
how different everything
looks with these glasses.

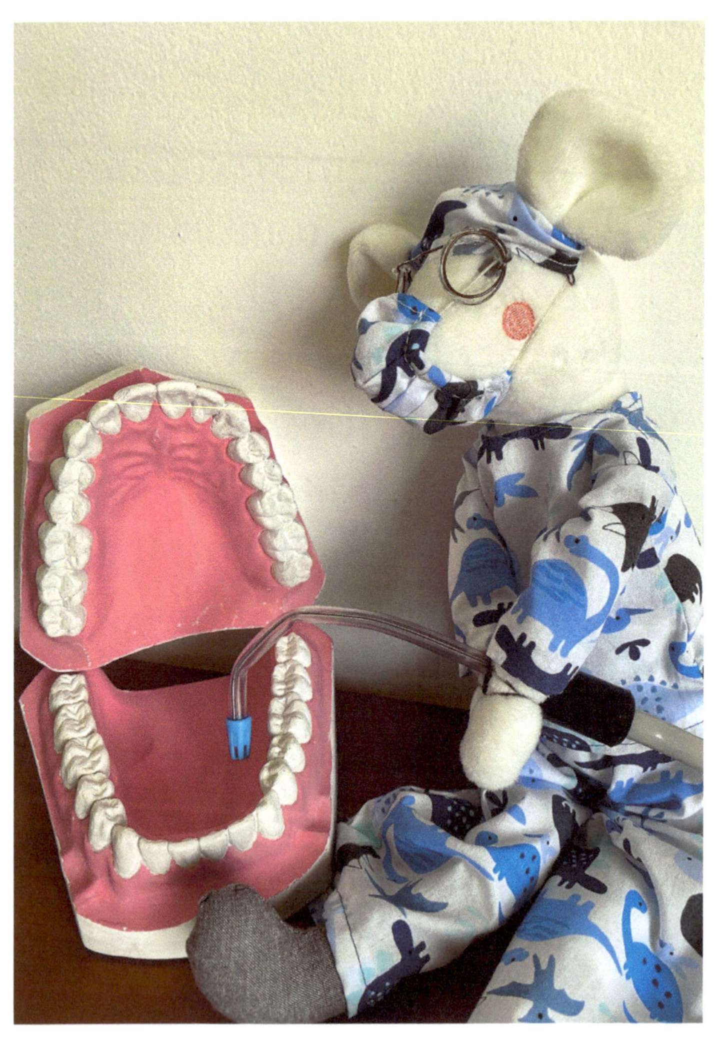

38

Your dentist
has a straw called an "ejector"
that does the opposite
function: it removes saliva
and water from your mouth
to make the cleaning
process more comfortable.

Santiago Mouse
is showing you that
it is so easy to hold.

You will be able
to do it sometimes.

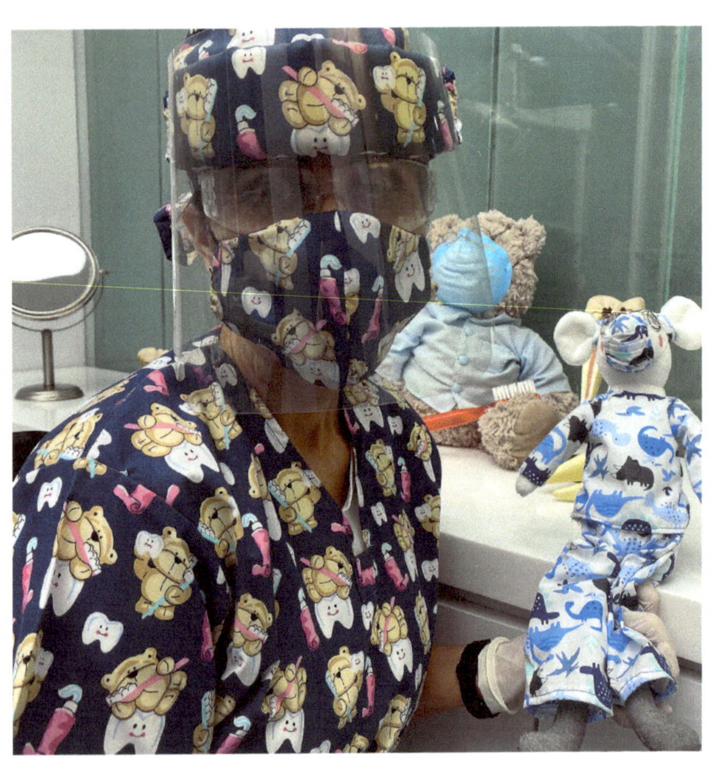

Sometimes
going to the dentist
can be a "bit annoying",
but it should NEVER be
a painful experience.
For example, if Genaro Bear
leaned on your shoulder
after a minute, you would say,
"Uff! How annoying!
This is equivalent
to the discomfort of
removing cavities".

**Tell the dentist if you
feel discomfort or pain!
It's important to tell
the dentist how and
what you are feeling.**

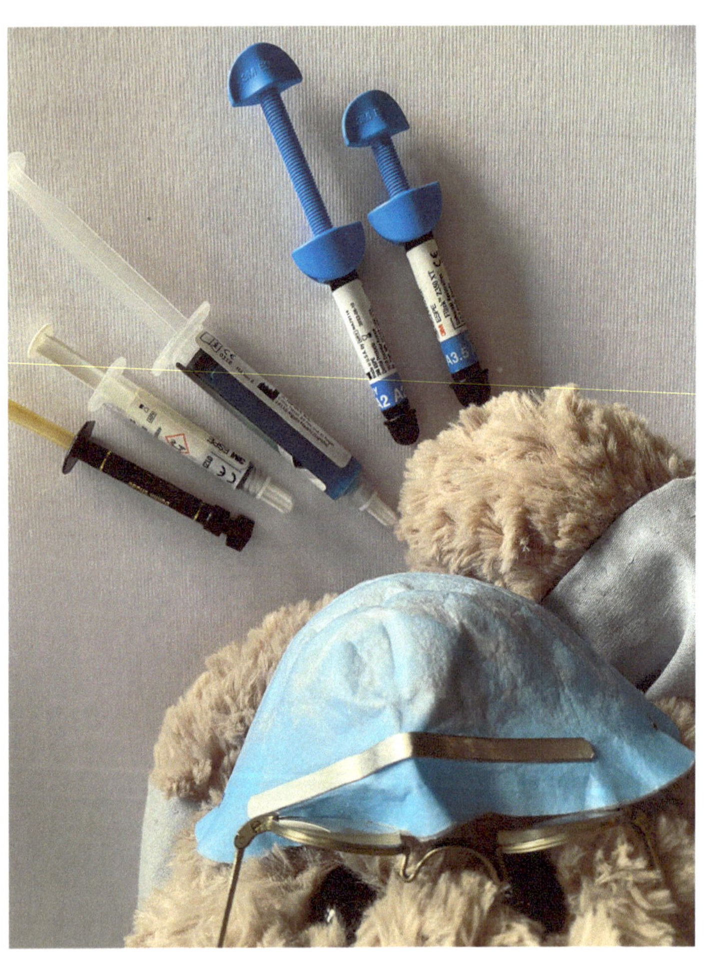

Dentists also use tools
that can be scary,
such as syringes.

However, you should
know that the ones
your dentist uses DO NOT
have needles.

They are used to place
small amounts of material on
your teeth.

You can always ask your
dentist to show you the tools,
so that you are not scared.

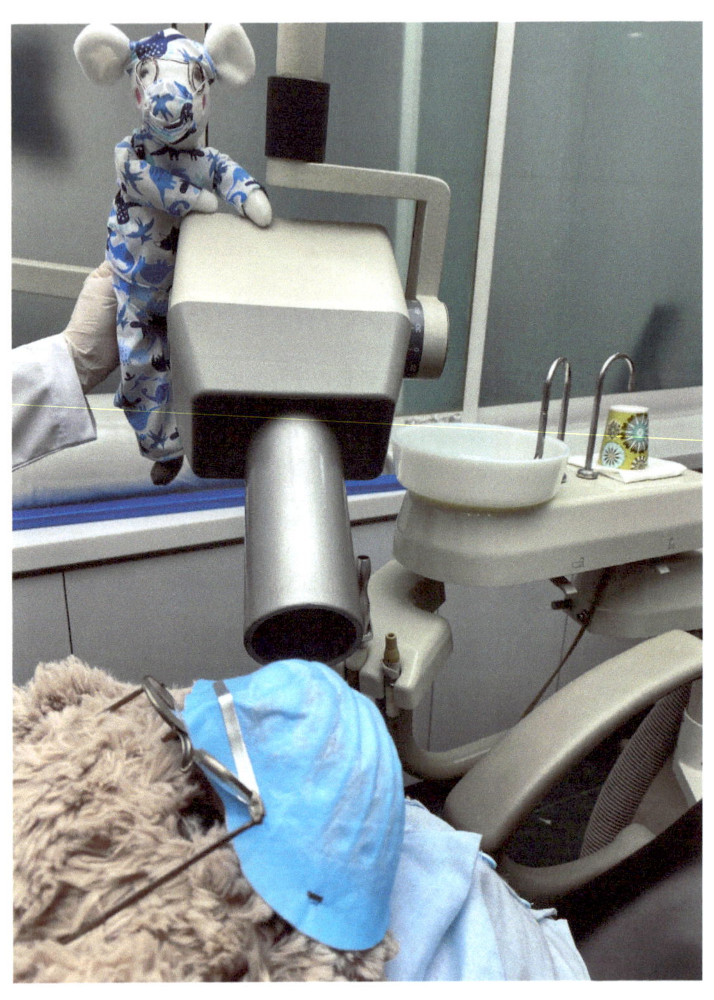

Santiago Mouse
reminds you that
if you go too long without
brushing your teeth,
many cavities,
even large ones can appear.

Your dentist will need
to take an X-ray.

**Such an
interesting word!**

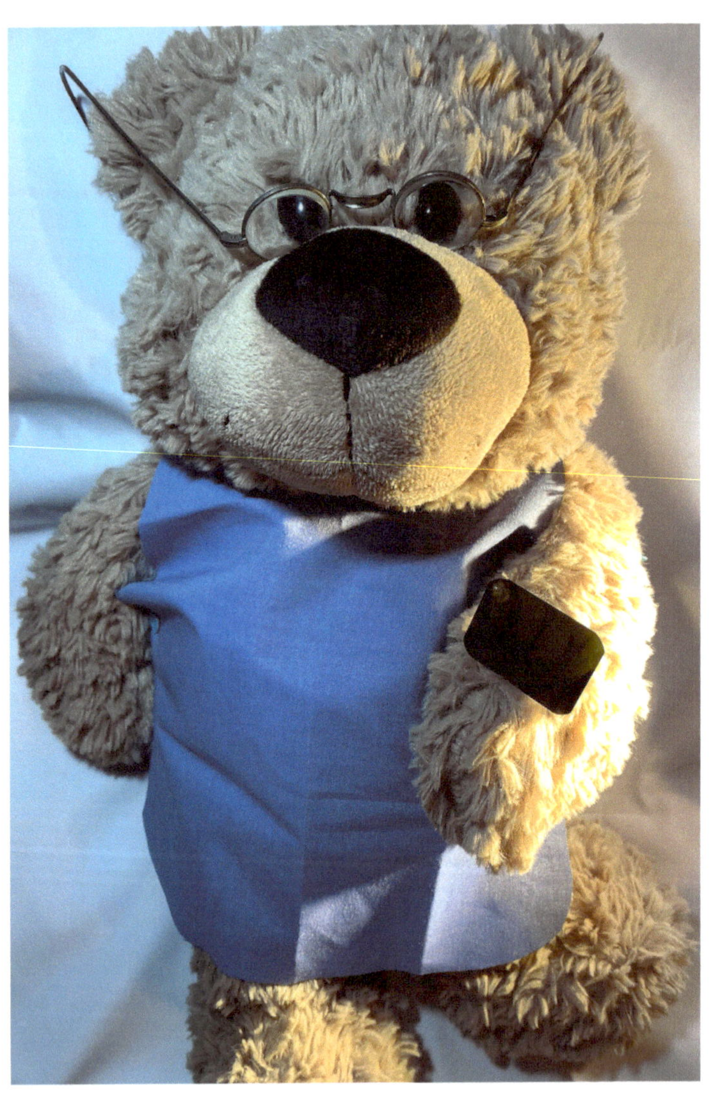

46

X-rays;
This means
that the dentist will take
a special black and white
photo of your
teeth and bones.

You'll have to wear a heavy
apron to protect you from
the light that comes out of
the device as if it were a very
effective sunscreen.

Just like Genaro Bear
is wearing.

D5
D4
D3
D2
UPPER
D2
D3
D6
D6
E5
E4
E3
LEFT
E2
E2
RIGHT
E3
E4
E5
E6
D4
D3
D2
LOWER
D2
D3
D4
D5
E4
E3
E2
E2
E3
E4
E5

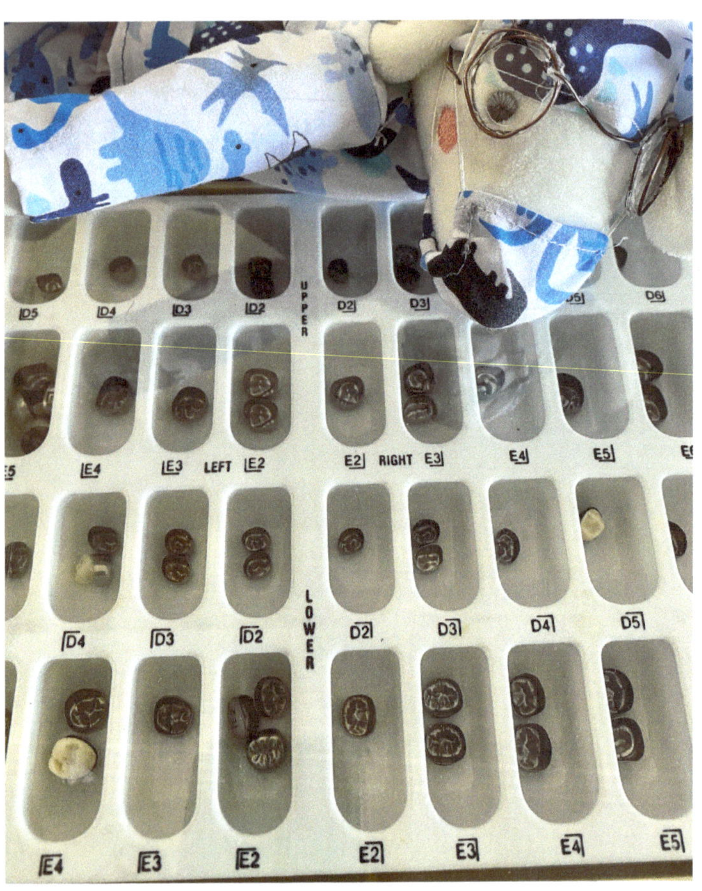

48

There are times
when your molar is so
badly damaged that
the dentist needs to put
a crown on it.
It may sound like royalty,
but in reality, it is like a
Knight's Armor since your
tooth is fragile, and we
have to protect it.

**With your crown,
you can continue
chewing everything
you like!**

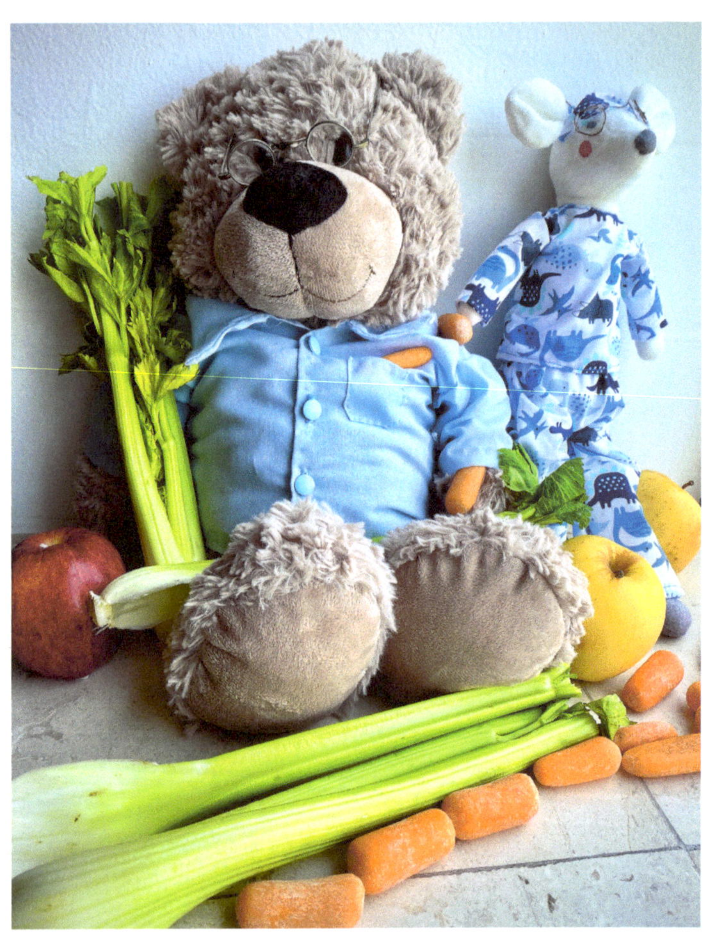

Genaro Bear, Santiago Mouse
and your dentist recommend
you to eat apples, carrots,
and celery, as they help keep
your teeth clean and healthy.

It is preferable not to chew
gum or candy and always
brush your teeth very well
to grow up to an adult with
a healthy and bright smile.

**Now you know
everything you'll need
to make the next visit
to your dentist a new
and fun adventure!**

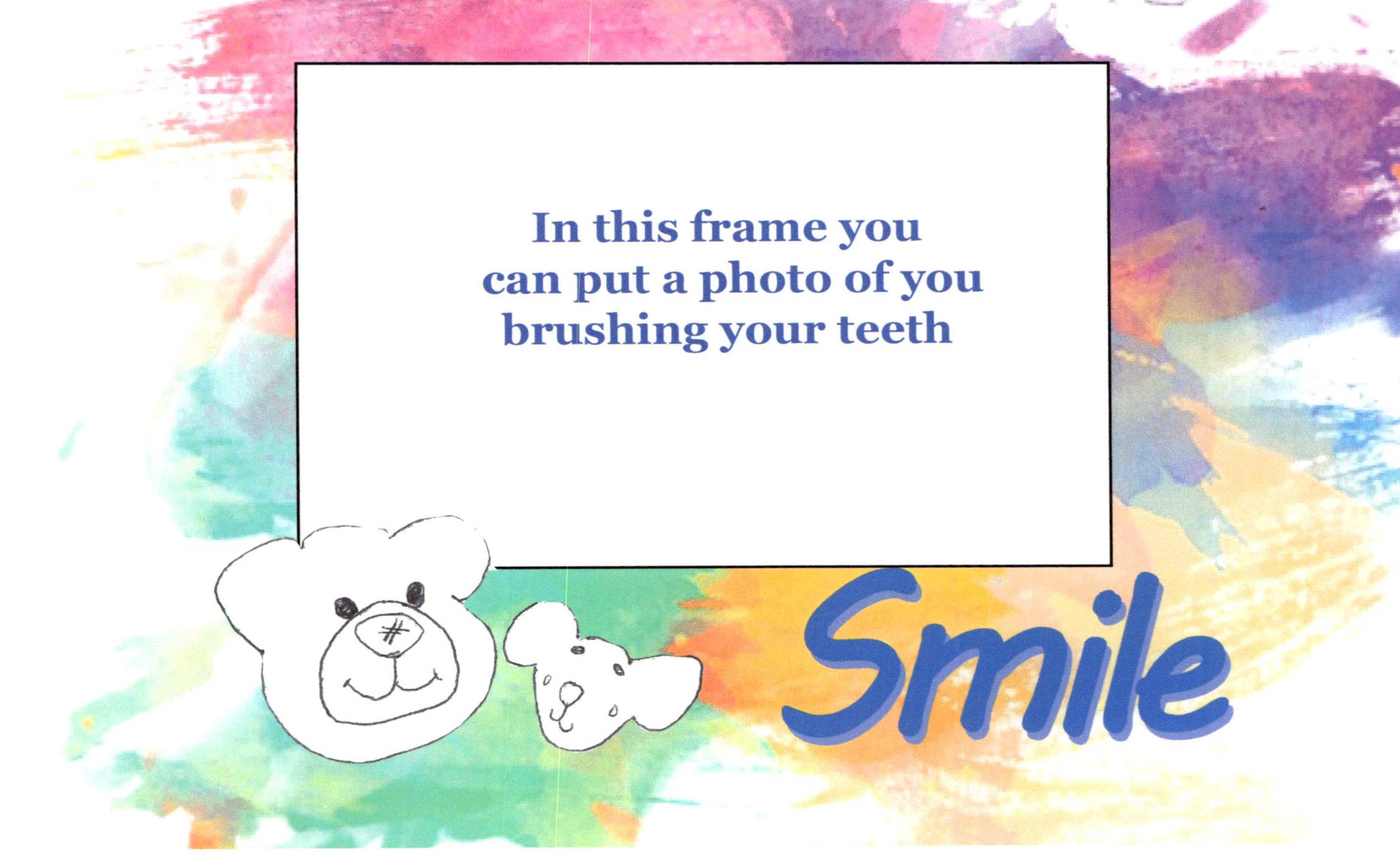

In this frame you
can put a photo of you
brushing your teeth
Smile

Cut out, drawn in, have fun, and remember
to brush your teeth thoroughly.

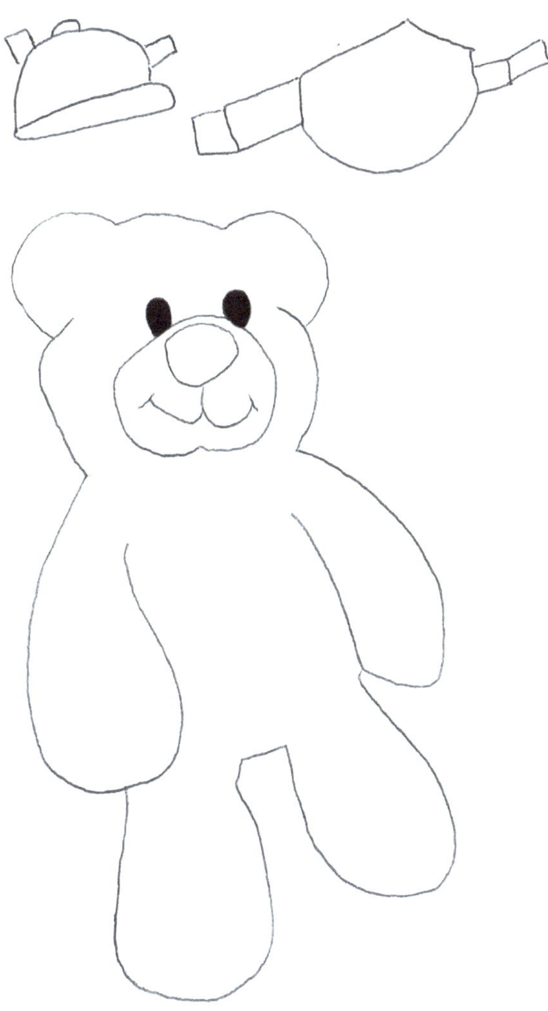

**Cut out, drawn in, have fun, and remember
to brush your teeth thoroughly.**

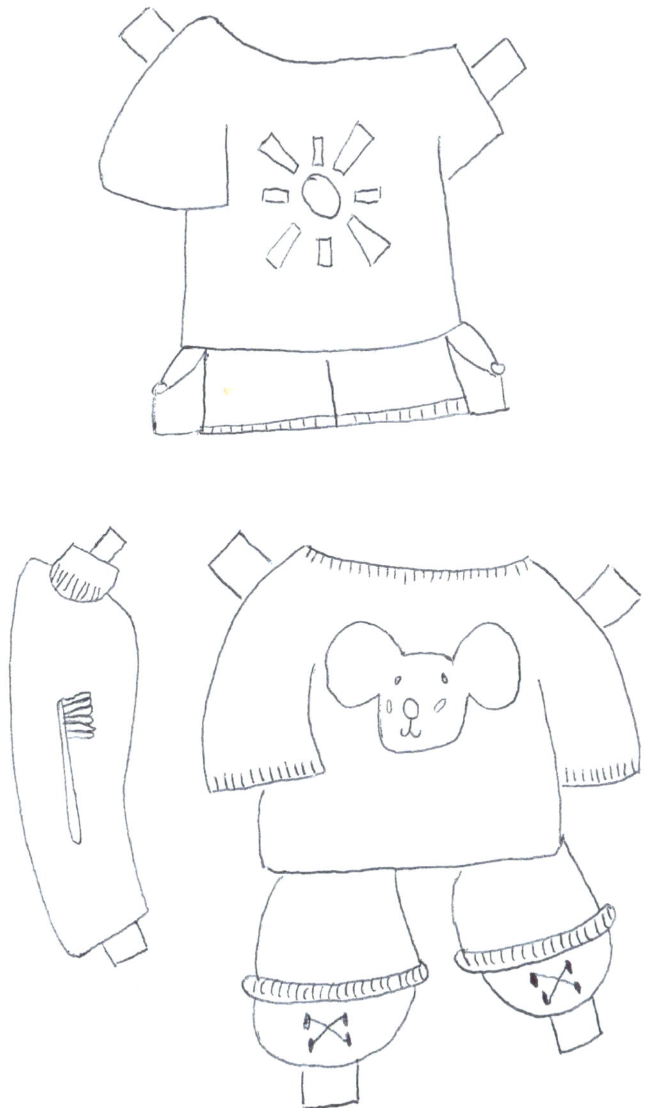

Cut out, drawn in, have fun, and remember to brush your teeth thoroughly.

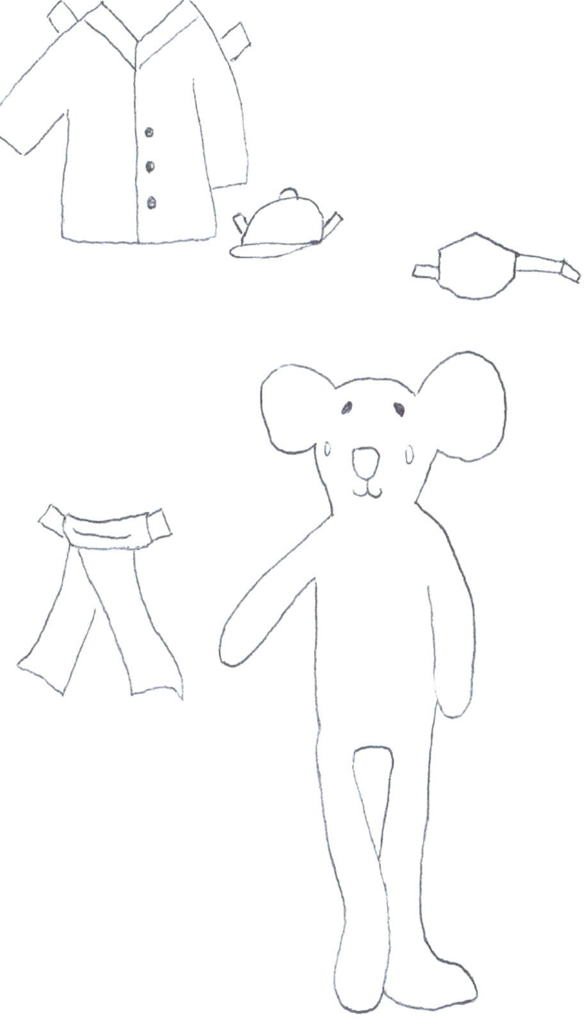

Cut out, drawn in, have fun, and remember to brush your teeth thoroughly.

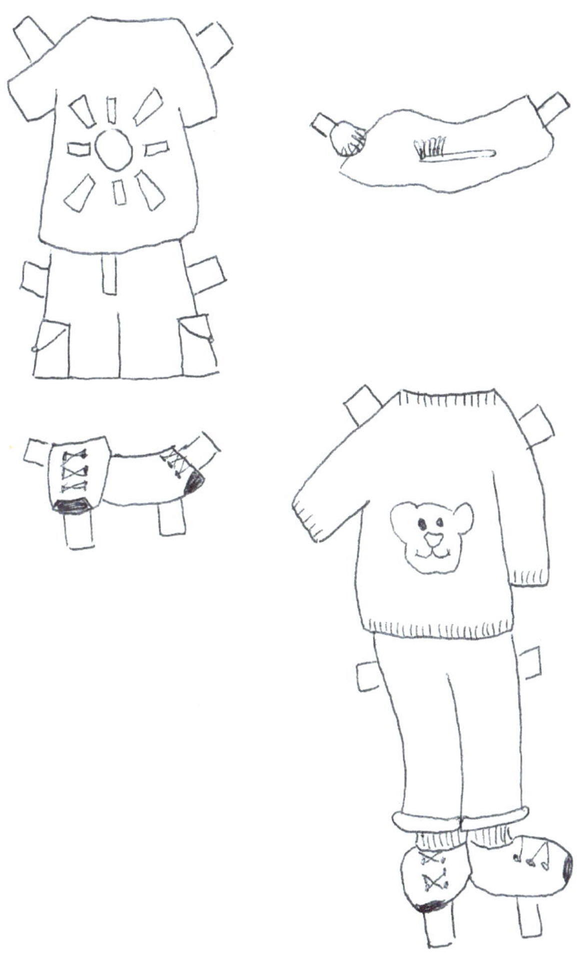